The Healthy Meal Prep Cookbook

The nutritional guide with weekly food programs with ready meals. Cook the best foods to live healthily without sacrificing flavors.

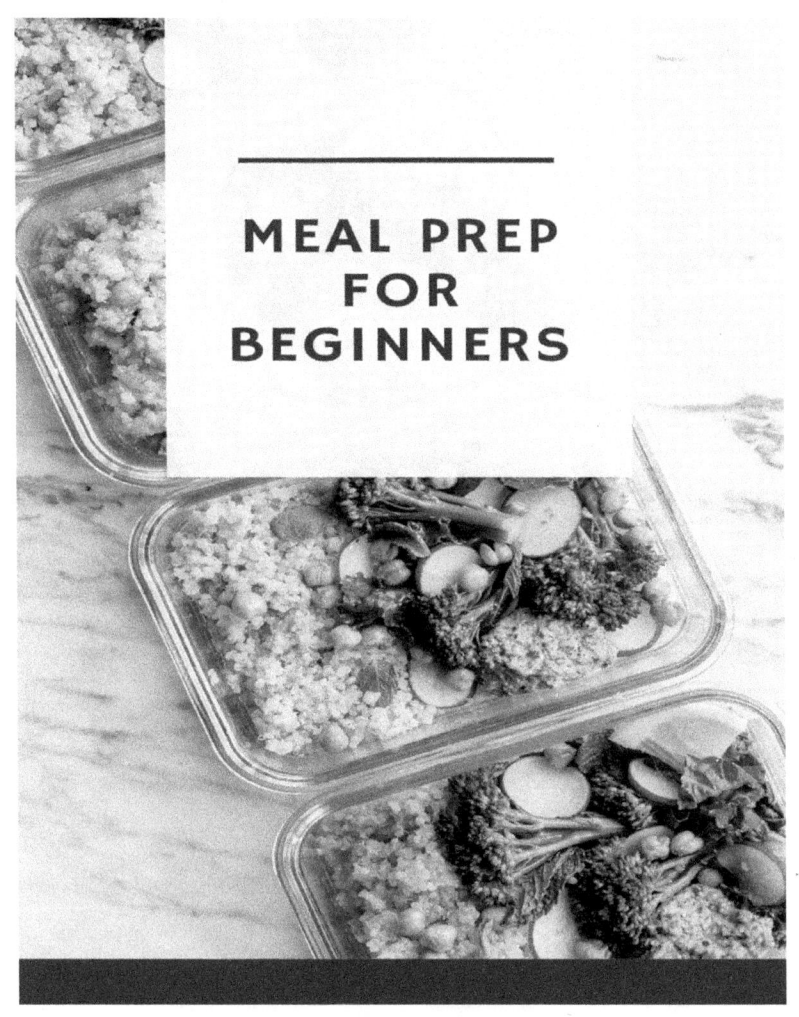

MEAL PREP FOR BEGINNERS

COPYRIGHT

© Copyright 2019 all right reserved by DAVE FILL

This document is geared towards providing exact and reliable information with regard to the topic and issue covered. The publication is sold with the idea that the publisher is not required to render accounting, officially permitted or otherwise qualified services. If advice is necessary, legal or professional, a practiced individual in the profession should be ordered.

- From a Declaration of Principles which was accepted and approved equally by a Committee of the American Bar Association and a Committee of Publishers and Associations.

In no way is it legal to reproduce, duplicate, or transmit any part of this document in either electronic means or in printed format. Recording of this publication is strictly prohibited, and any storage of this document is not allowed unless with written permission from the publisher. All rights reserved.

The information provided herein is stated to be truthful and consistent, in that any liability, in terms of inattention or otherwise, by any usage or abuse of any policies, processes, or directions contained within is the solitary and utter responsibility of the recipient reader. Under no circumstances will any legal responsibility or blame be held against the publisher for any reparation, damages, or monetary loss due to the information herein, either directly or indirectly.

Respective authors own all copyrights not held by the publisher.

The information herein is offered for informational purposes solely and is universal as so. The presentation of the information is without contract or any type of guarantee assurance.

Table of CONTENTS

COPYRIGHT 5

INTRODUCTION 10

WHAT YOU SHOULD KNOW ABOUT MEAL PREP 14
- WHAT IS MEAL PREP? 15
- FOR WHAT REASON SHOULD YOU MEAL PREP? 17
- IS MEAL PREP FOR EVERYONE? 18
- WHAT FOODS CAN I MEAL PREP? 20
- THE MOST EFFECTIVE METHOD TO GET STARTED WITH MEAL PREP 29

SIGNIFICANT BENEFITS OF MEAL PREP 44
- FOUR KEYS TO SUCCESSFUL MEAL PREP 59

A HELPFUL HEALTHY EATING STRATEGY 62

STEP BY STEP TIPS TO START A MEAL PREP 70

EXTREME GRAB-AND-GO BREAKFASTS YOU CAN MEAL-PREP 79
- AVOCADO AND EGG BREAKFAST MEAL PREP 88
- BANANA AND CHOCOLATE CHIP PREPARED OATMEAL CUPS 91
- EGG BISCUITS WITH HAM, KALE, AND CAULIFLOWER RICE 96

THINGS I ALWAYS DO WHEN MEAL PREPPING 100

THINGS I WISH SOMEONE TOLD ME BEFORE I STARTED MEAL PREPPING 104

INTRODUCTION

If you resemble numerous individuals, you moan at the idea of doing meal prep. While you realize it is something you have to do, it doesn't mean you like it! Meal prep requires some serious energy, yet if you take a gander at preparing state your vegetables only once for the entire week, then you will think that its simpler to eat healthy home-prepared meals each night. A few nourishments, a few vegetables are anything but difficult to prepare early and spare well. There are steps you can take with your meal wanting to make the errand simpler and afterward you will discover you invest less energy doing the meal prep and additional time making the most of your nourishment!

Give us a chance to take a gander at a couple of meal-prep thoughts...

1. One Recipe, Many Variations. Maybe the most significant tedious assignment with meal prep is attempting to make sense of what to cook in any case. You need to chase down plans, make sense of what will work with your weight loss abstain from food and afterward buy every one of some staple goods required. Tedious stuff!

Rather, take a gander at discovering one formula offering a few varieties. For example, you may make a vegetable pan fried food. You can simply modify the vegetables you put in the sautéed food, swap out the chicken for hamburger as wanted, and even change the sauce a bit. It is a similar meal by and large, however with little changes that ought to be sufficient to keep you keen on proceeding to continue with your weight loss diet plan.

The more you become acquainted with preparing a similar sort of meals again and again, the simpler it will be to design your meal prep out for the week.

2. Two Words: Slow Cooker. Slow cooking is excessively simple, and a technique for cooking everybody ought to get into doing now and again. Simply put every one of the fixings in the moderate cooker in the first part of the day, turn it on, and when you show up home from work, the nourishment will be prepared to serve. In addition, you can make a significantly estimated bunch, which implies you will eat healthy meals a few times during your week.

3. Purchase Pre-Chopped Vegetables. The last plan to consider is purchasing pre-slashed vegetables. Cutting up vegetables is often one employment individuals disdain doing the most, so make it simpler for yourself. Get them all set, so there is next to zero prep work included.

While you will pay somewhat more for pre-hacked vegetables, it is cash very much spent.

There you have a couple of thoughts to consider utilizing to help make meal prep simpler. If you pursue these tips, adhering to your weight loss diet will be simpler than any time in recent memory.

In spite of the fact that dealing with your ailment can be extremely testing, Type 2 diabetes isn't a condition you should simply live with. You can roll out basic improvements to your day by day schedule and lower both your weight and your glucose levels. Keep it together, the more you do it, the simpler it gets.

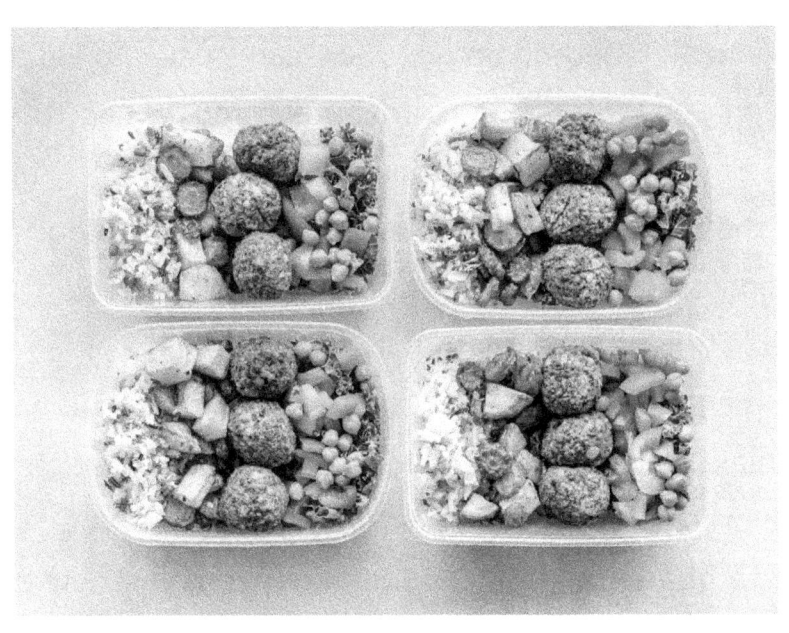

WHAT YOU SHOULD KNOW ABOUT MEAL PREP

Meal prep is in excess of a nourishment pattern: It's a convenient methodology you can use to make heavenly, hand crafted nourishment you'll need to eat each day — without the pause. And keeping in mind that the final products look amazing, meal prep doesn't require confused arranging or devices. All you truly need is time and real effort.

This manual for meal prep shows you all that you have to think about make-ahead meals — in addition to Bulletproof-accommodating methodologies you can take to guarantee your nourishment remains new and nutritious.

WHAT IS MEAL PREP?

Need to figure out how to meal prep? Cook and store impeccable make-ahead meals with this present fledgling's aide, in addition to get 10 plans to move.

Basically, meal prep implies prepping for meals. And keeping in mind that solitary serve meals are the most well-known way to deal with meal prep, there are different sorts to look over relying upon your timetable, tastes, and dietary needs.

Kinds of meal prep include:

Full make-ahead meals: You cook a whole meal and store it in your ice chest or cooler.

Clump cooking or solidifying: Make various meals, then segment and store them. This methodology is helpful for plans you can without much of a stretch cook in huge sums (like enormous pots of soup, rice, or crushed sweet potatoes).

Meals for one: Prepare nourishment and segment it in single-serving holders. (Normally enough to last a couple of days.)

Fixing prep: For individuals who like to prepare and serve nourishment at the same time, just prep parts of plans. Hack veggies, blend flavors, or marinade meat ahead of time to spare time when you're prepared to cook.

For what reason should you meal prep?

Figuring out how to meal prep will spare you time, yet it additionally sets aside cash and diminishes squander. What's more, not normal for handled meals, this strategy gives you complete power over what goes in your nourishment — ideal for any individual who needs to remain on track with their health objectives.

Is meal prep for everyone?

Need to figure out how to meal prep? Cook and store flawless make-ahead meals with this current apprentice's guide, in addition to get 10 plans to motivate.

Meal prep can profit individuals viewing their macros or attempting to chop down their cook time during the week. Be that as it may, a few types of meal prep may not be for everybody.

When you prepare and store your meals, they may mature sufficiently long to cause a negative response. How? When stuffed and put away, extra nourishment can discharge histamines as a side-effect of the maturation procedure. If you're especially delicate to these aggravates, your remains could cause mind mist and exhaustion.

Since everybody's histamine resistance is different, it's as yet justified, despite all the trouble to attempt meal prep, maintain a strategic distance from high-histamine nourishments when you cook, and check whether the procedure works for you. Consider meal prepping for a shorter time span, or prepping single fixings rather than full meals.

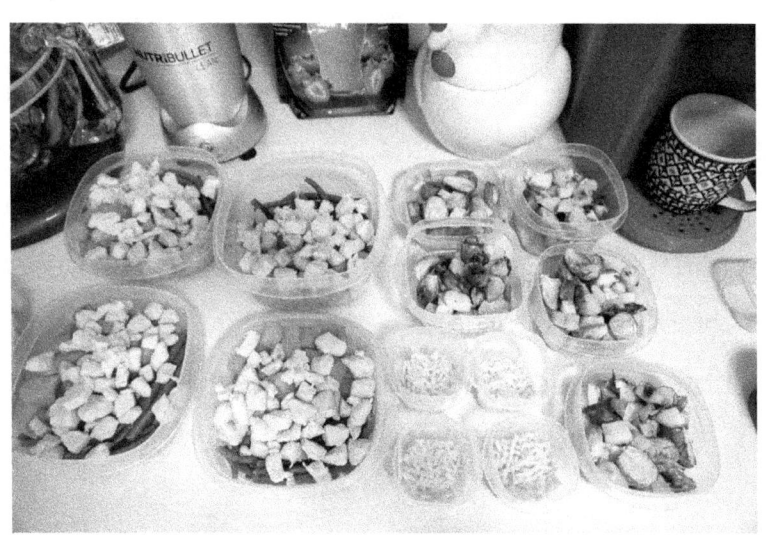

What foods can i meal prep?

Need to figure out how to meal prep? Cook and store immaculate make-ahead meals with this present tenderfoot's guide, in addition to get 10 plans to motivate.

You can meal prep any nourishment that holds up well away and tastes satisfactory to you following a couple of days in the cooler. Cooked meat, simmered vegetables, soups, sauces, nuts, and stiff crude vegetables make great bases for meal prep plans.

Yet, you can't meal prep everything. Delicate vegetables, cut organic product, and crunchy nourishment like saltines will just get gentler in your icebox — settling on them less perfect decisions for meal prep.

If you're new to meal prep, consider how you'll warm nourishment. Will you just approach a microwave at mealtime, or would you be able to utilize a stovetop or broiler? Consider plans that you can appreciate cold or tenderly warm so you don't hazard harming fats and proteins in your nourishment.

Above all, pick plans that you as of now appreciate extra and can cook effortlessly. Then you can stretch out with new plans and nourishment pairings. Keep it easy to begin so you don't wind up squandering nourishment.

The most effective method to MEAL PREP: FIRST STEPS Need to figure out how to meal prep? Cook and store impeccable make-ahead meals with this present learner's guide, in addition to get 10 plans to motivate.

GET HIGH-QUALITY FOOD STORAGE CONTAINERS

Utilize quality nourishment stockpiling compartments to keep meal prep nourishment hot (or cold). Warm, tempered steel holders are the perfect answer for keeping nourishment warm or chilled, and arrive in an assortment of sizes. You can refrigerate them early or warm them with bubbling water before adding cold or hot nourishments to make them last considerably more. China is the most secure arrangement of all, as long as you plan on making the most of your meal cold and can deal with it cautiously.

Reusable plastics and plastic sacks are never prescribed for pressing meal prep nourishments. Beside cancer-causing BPA, even non-BPA plastics can contain estrogenic chemicals that drain into your nourishment and disturb your hormones. Furthermore, if you heat these plastics in the microwave, you're likewise adding radiation to the blend. Abstain from putting away nourishment in plastic whenever you can to keep your meal prep dishes ideal.

Pick Recipes And Build Your Menu

With basic plans close by, choose what you'll cook for the week and timetable the times of the week when you need to make the most of your meals. Consider what you requirement for those plans, in addition to any missing basics you need (like flavors or ghee), and make your staple rundown.

Calendar TIME FOR MEAL PREP

You can't meal prep without prep time. Calendar a window one to two days of the week to prep your meals. If you perform multiple tasks a bit (utilize your broiler and stove top to prep more than one nourishment on the double, for instance), you'll cut down on time considerably more.

Oat Milk Is the Newest Non-Dairy Darling. In any case, Is It Nutritious?

Is Nutmeg Safe? What You Should Know About This Holiday Spice

What are Macros, and Should You Count Them?

Step by step instructions to Do an Elimination Diet, and Why Everyone Needs to Do One

Step by step instructions to MEAL PREP: FOOD SAFETY

Need to figure out how to meal prep? Cook and store immaculate make-ahead meals with this current learner's guide, in addition to get 10 plans to move.

There are no firm rules for to what extent your nourishment will remain new. The wellbeing of your meal prep depends a ton on your icebox, how you stuffed it, and the nature of your fixings.

Start with the FDA's rules for ice chest and cooler stockpiling to illuminate to what extent you can store meal prep nourishments, and practice presence of mind when you pack nourishment so it can last more. Utilize isolated compartments to dodge cross-pollution (or flavor tainting), and pack wet nourishment separate from dry nourishment. Use ice packs to keep cold dishes cold, and pre-warmed protected holders to keep hot nourishments hot. Furthermore, obviously, clean your hands and produce before you cook.

Most meal prep meals will last between 3-5 days in the ice chest. If you need to meal prep for the entire week, you'll need to plan two days per week to do as such, (for example, Sunday and Wednesday) to keep nourishment as new as could reasonably be expected.

Would it be advisable for me to MEAL PREP IF I DON'T LIKE EATING THE SAME THING EVERY DAY?

Prepping precisely the same meal consistently can spare a great deal of time — however it additionally gets exhausting. If you feel burnt out on eating similar meals again and again, make little changes to your meal prep to make each dish somewhat different. For instance, swap in different veggies, sauces, or enhancements for every compartment to keep things fascinating.

On the other hand, you can prep and stop different plans early. Then, defrost a couple of holders in the icebox consistently so you can appreciate different dishes consistently.

The most effective method to MEAL PREP: AVOIDING COMMON MISTAKES

Need to figure out how to meal prep? Cook and store flawless make-ahead meals with this present apprentice's guide, in addition to get 10 plans to motivate.

KEEP MEAL PREP SIMPLE

For beginners, start straightforward. Make one-pot plans or spotlight on one primary dish, and maintain a strategic distance from the compulsion to go through an entire day preparing elaborate meals. Such a large number of plans can entangle your meal prep quick, and you might not have any desire to do it again if it was too hard the first run through. Have a go at making only one formula early, then meal prep extra dishes when you get settled.

PREP BALANCED MEALS

Contingent upon your eating regimen and health objectives, plan meals that will keep you fulfilled. It's anything but difficult to make a major bowl of bean stew for lunch, however it wouldn't fill in as a total meal for a great many people. Ensure you get enough of the correct nutrition classes to round out your macros.

COOK RECIPES YOU'LL ACTUALLY EAT

For whatever length of time that your meal prep dishes are adjusted, you don't have to fan out of your customary range of familiarity. For beginners, make plans you realize you'll adore — anything less could bring about squandered nourishment (and sat around idly).

MAKE ENOUGH FOOD

Ensure you prep enough nourishment to accommodate your arrangement. Besides, remember your timetable — occasions from work snacks to glad hours can meddle with mealtime, so foresee whether you genuinely need to meal prep consistently.

MEAL PREP IDEAS: 10 RECIPES WORTH TRYING

Need to figure out how to meal prep? Cook and store impeccable make-ahead meals with this current novice's guide, in addition to get 10 plans to motivate. Prepared to attempt meal prep? Get roused with these plans:

Sweet potato curry with cilantro lime cauliflower rice

Purple squashed cauliflower

Chicken soup

Bacon pineapple shrimp sticks

Thai marinated skirt steak

Slow cooker mexican destroyed meat

Rosemary bagels

Thyme and zucchini wastes

Shaved Brussels grows serving of mixed greens with lemon thyme vinaigrette (pack vinaigrette independently)

Vanilla turmeric fat bombs

If you're keen on less-wild mealtimes, sparing time in the kitchen or settling on healthier nourishment decisions, you have to attempt meal prepping. Meal prep can run from basically preparing cooler smoothie packs for breakfast to preparing total suppers for the forthcoming week. There is nobody right way or technique to meal prep—it's about what works best for you. What's more, you don't have to spend your whole Sunday in the kitchen to complete it. In any event, spending as meager as 30 minutes arranging and prepping meals will make it simpler to eat well during the week.

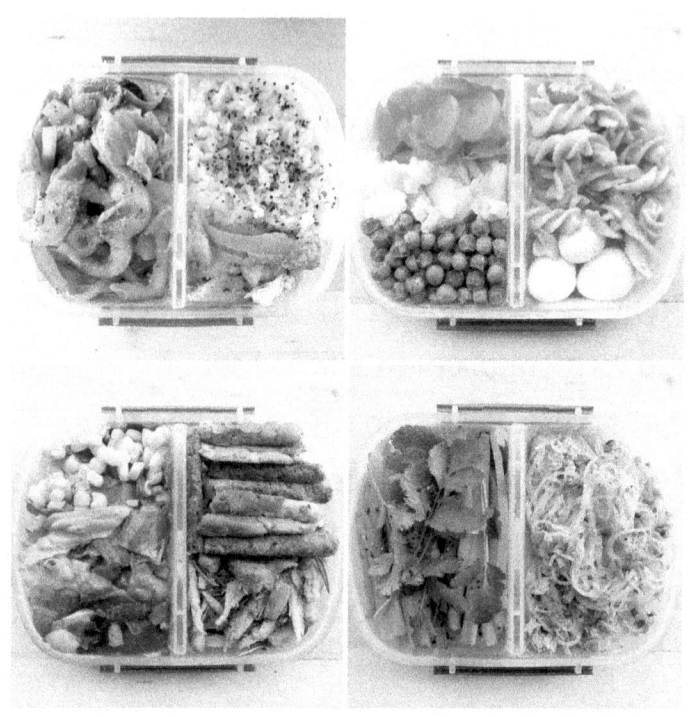

The most effective method to Get Started with Meal Prep

Peruse these straightforward strides to make sense of how to begin with meal prep.

Stage 1: Determine the Best Prep Method for You
Contingent upon your calendar, the meals you like to prep ahead, and your cooking style, one (or a blend) of these meal-prep techniques may work best for you:

Make-ahead meals: For those with brief period to prepare meals during the week, cooking total meals ahead of time to be warmed at mealtimes (like a pot of soup or a goulash) makes for very quick weeknight suppers.

Group cooking/solidifying: Batch cooking is preparing numerous bunches of a formula to be administered out and solidified for meals in the weeks to come. For instance, multiplying a bean stew formula or steaming additional rice to stop and use in the following three to a half year.

Separately divided meals: Those with specific health objectives or searching for the comfort of get and-go meals may decide to prepare nourishments and bit them into singular servings. Think medium-term oats partitioned into single-serving compartments, and artisan container plates of mixed greens.

Prepared to-cook fixings: If you want to prepare meals directly before serving, prepping fixings (e.g., slashing onion and peppers ahead of time for bean stew) eliminates kitchen time, which can be particularly useful on a bustling weeknight.

Stage 2: Make a Plan

When you've settled on the type(s) of meal prep you'd advantage most from, put in no time flat making a basic course of action to keep you sorted out. Consider the accompanying as you compose a menu and prep plan:

Pick meal(s) to prep: Are you hoping to streamline your morning schedule? Prepping smoothie packs eliminates time spent on breakfast. If occupied nights limit time to cook during the week, consider make-ahead meals that can be effectively warmed.

Compose your menu: When arranging your menu and prep, depend on some time tested plans that you've cooked previously, with a couple of new plans tossed in. Keeping things basic will help spare you time. Construct meals around regular produce for best flavor and worth think butternut squash in the fall and ready summer tomatoes. If you don't know where to begin, a cluster of dark colored rice, a couple of chicken bosoms and a plate of simmered vegetables are effectively collected into everything from rice bowls to singed rice to servings of mixed greens.

Calendar your prep: Setting aside some time for really prepping is significant! Consider meal prepping around the same time you shop and compose a sensible prep plan. It may not be sensible to prepare five meals in 60 minutes, however you may have the opportunity to prep certain elements for the plans. Also, if you like a test, set a clock to keep you on task!

Stage 3: Take Stock and Shop

With your menu arranged, it's a great opportunity to assemble a shopping list. In any case, before racing to the market, take stock of your kitchen.

Load up on staples: Stocking your wash room with an assortment of solid products like dried herbs and flavor mixes and rack stable entire grains like dark colored rice and quinoa-simplifies meal prepping. Low-sodium canned beans and soup, ice chest staples like eggs and precooked chicken wiener, and a couple of cooler benevolent nourishments can change prepped fixings into meals in minutes. You can even put together your whole meal plan with respect to storeroom staples, as in this 7-Day Pantry Staples Dinner Plan.

Manufacture a superior shopping list: Navigate the supermarket rapidly with a rundown sorted out by office. Keep a running stock of nourishments you every now and again use during week by week prep, similar to olive oil, onions or darker rice, and add these to your rundown when important.

Check your stockpile of holders: Depending on your arrangement for the week, you will require a combination of capacity compartments, including glass and plastic holders with covers and zip-top stockpiling and cooler sacks. Consider these holder proposals for pressing work snacks.

Stage 4: Prep and Store

We've made it to the fun part-start prepping your meals! Here are some useful hints to remember before you start cleaving:

Benefit as much as possible from your time: Begin with nourishments that require the longest cooking occasions. Preheat the broiler and prepare fixings that will be cooked first. Heat water to the point of boiling for longer-cooking grains like farro or darker rice. If two plans require a similar fixing, as slashed onions, prep the onions for the two plans on the double, then partition to use as required. To spare the progression of expecting to wash your cutting board between assignments, cut produce that will be eaten crude first, trailed by produce to be cooked. Continuously make sure to utilize a perfect cutting board and utensils subsequent to preparing crude proteins, similar to meat or poultry.

Be aware of capacity life: If put away in hermetically sealed compartments, cut vegetables like onions and peppers will keep for a few days in the fridge. Heartier vegetables, as slashed carrots and winter squash, will keep for in any event four days. Lettuce and greens that have been washed, dried and kept in the icebox can remain crisp for as long as seven days. Cooked vegetables, grains and dishes containing meat, poultry, fish or eggs ought to be expended inside three to four days, and make certain to warm these to 165°F.

Stop appropriately for best quality: Foods like soups, stews, dishes and cooked grains are effectively solidified for future meals. During those insane occupied weeks, there is nothing more gratifying than dismantling a prepared to-warm meal from the cooler! For soups and cooked grains, cool to room temperature (inside 2 hours) and store in quart-size plastic holders or zip-top cooler packs. Leave an inch at the highest point of holders for nourishment to extend as it solidifies. Top meals with wax paper and spread firmly in foil. Name and date compartments, and set suggestions to devour solidified nourishments inside three to a half year. Make certain to warm to a cooking temperature of 165°F when prepared to serve.

Stage 5: Enjoy the Fruits (and Vegetables) of Your Labor

With a touch of training, you will find a style of meal prep that works best for you. Regardless of whether you prep elements for one meal, prepare work snacks for the week, or cook a twofold bunch of stew to solidify for one month from now, any measure of time spent meal prepping yields enormous returns. If you're needing menu motivation, look at our library of meal plans and discover one that works best for you.

We would all be able to concur that creation healthy decisions when eating out, or eating out regularly as a rule, can get expensive rapidly. However, with meal prepping, you are allowed to pick and eat nourishments that suit your health objectives, without leaving an imprint in your wallet.

Be that as it may, before you get into the healthy act of meal prepping, here are a few things you should know.

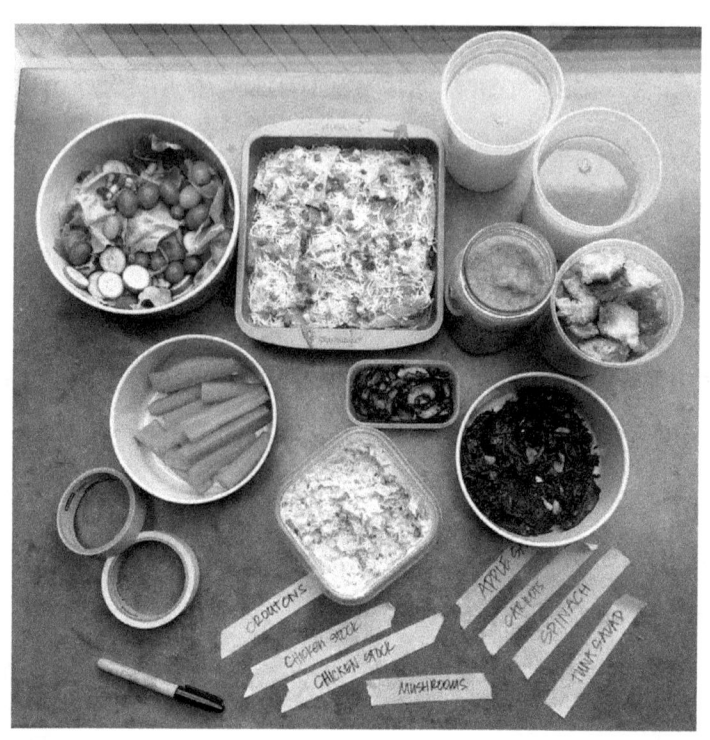

1. Know why you need to meal prep

Meal prepping is the act of preparing nourishment ahead of time to last you all through a range of time, normally seven days. It's an extraordinary path for occupied honey bees to pick healthy, hand crafted meals while setting aside time and cash. There are numerous motivations to meal prep, yet by a wide margin the most prevalent are the accompanying:

To accomplish wellness objectives (picking up muscle, getting more fit, or both)

To eliminate costs by planning meals

To spare time and not need to consider what to eat constantly

Knowing your very own purpose behind selecting to meal prep will make it simpler to focus on the procedure over the long haul!

2. Try not to attempt to meal prep for the entire week on your first attempt

Does the idea of meal prepping all of a sudden make your palms sweat-soaked? Slow your roll. As a beginning, prepare only a couple of day of meals. The first run through is consistently the most testing, yet simply keep at it and soon you'll have the option to do this in your rest.

3. There's no disgrace in pre-cooked/pre-cut fixings

Who has an opportunity to prepare, marinate and heat chicken without any preparation? If you're lacking in time, simply go for a locally acquired choice for meats, and perhaps incorporate pre-washed and pre-cut vegetables. Loading up on these staple things spares you a lot of prep time. Grocery store rotisserie chicken, plate of mixed greens, and solidified natural products are for the most part similarly as great.

4. Realize that not all meals should be cooked

Prepping a meal doesn't imply that each and every dish needs to go into a broiler or over a stove. A basic verdant plate of mixed greens for lunch or supper, or having organic product as a bite still falls under the umbrella of meal prepping. Indeed, even granola is promptly accessible and comes in different flavors, so as of now illuminates your morning meal and nibble hardships.

5. Put resources into high caliber hermetically sealed holders

Since meal prepping includes putting away nourishment for a few days, the nature of your nourishment compartments is a vital factor. You will require compartments that are comparative in size to your meals, and some littler holders for snacks. Costly nourishment compartments are not your lone alternative, however if your spending limit takes into account them, you should go for a great brand like Rubbermade. Having said that, any holder that can keep your meals new will do. Simply ensure that they're microwave-sheltered and simple to clean.

6. Make a rundown of dishes you need to prep

Make your life simpler by sorting out your meal prep routine and plan for advance. The initial step is to attempt to identify your own objectives. If you're attempting to get more fit, form muscle or set aside cash, search for plans that fit your day by day caloric and wholesome prerequisites.

Likewise ask yourself inquiries like 'how much time do I need to meal prep?' and 'Which fixings are promptly accessible in my nearby general store?' This will make it simpler to make and adhere to a shopping list for basic food item day.

7. Keep in mind, effortlessness is vital

Meal prepping isn't a challenge — you don't really need to reproduce the extravagant dishes you see on another person's Instagram account. If you have the certainty, time, and capacity to prepare eatery commendable meals, then definitely, let your abilities free! Be that as it may, for those of us who can just deal with the rudiments, having section level meal prep capacity is not the slightest bit a reason for concern.

To make your preparation much simpler, utilize comparable fixings on all or the vast majority of the dishes. A most loved element for meal preppers is broiled chicken, as this can be added to servings of mixed greens, sandwiches, or even as the primary dish. Get inventive by utilizing different plans and flavors to keep meals from getting excessively exhausting.

7. Set a day to shop and prep

To begin on the correct foot with meal prepping, set a specific date — ideally an end of the week — to do your shopping for food and preparing. Simply don't worry yourself! Meal prepping veterans for the most part recommend Sundays, as you will have plentiful time to concentrate on meal prepping without work and different duties disrupting everything.

8. Put resources into a moderate cooker

Slow cookers are the ideal hardware for individuals who are too eager to even think about standing by the stove and trust that their nourishment will be finished. These culinary terrible young men are excessively simple to utilize: you simply need to dump every one of the fixings in the moderate cooker pot and afterward set the clock and temperature. In only a couple of hours, you will have a steaming hot meal prepared with almost no exertion. If this thought stimulates your pickle, then putting resources into a moderate cooker will be a savvy move.

9. Remain motivated through online journals and YouTube

There are such a large number of wellness masters online who love sharing new and energizing meal prepping plans. What's more, if you have specific dietary prerequisites, you can likewise discover Youtubers that emphasis totally on specific eating regimens, for example, veggie lover, sans gluten, ketogenic, and numerous others — so whatever sort of diet you are following, you make certain to discover dishes that will be directly for you.

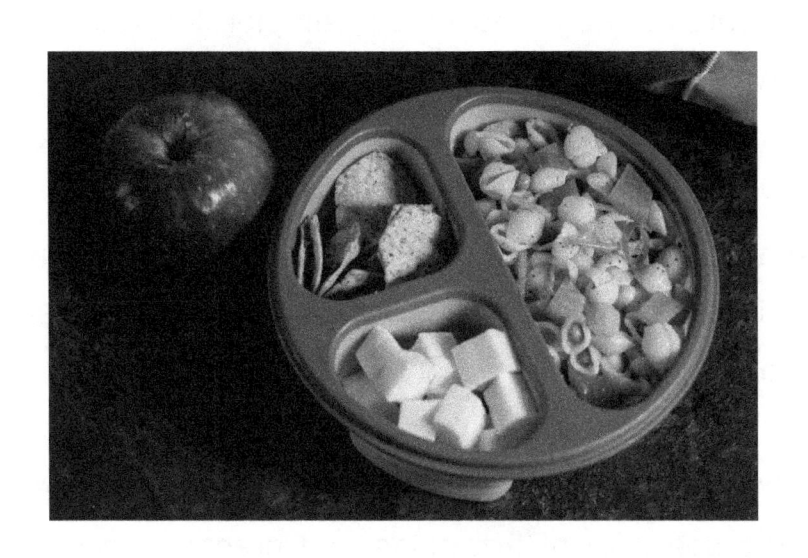

SIGNIFICANT BENEFITS OF MEAL PREP

Not prone to prepare? That might be a catastrophe waiting to happen.

Ever fantasize about how much simpler life would be if you were a snake with the goal that you'd just need to eat once every week? Simply consider constantly you'd spare every day not continually discovering plans, purchase staple goods, wash, hack and cook fixings, and tidy up a muddled kitchen. Nirvana, isn't that so?

The arrangement you're looking for is straightforward: meal prep. Rather than experiencing the exhausting day by day schedule recorded above, welcome into your life the specialty of arranging and preparing a few or the entirety of your meals ahead of time. This could mean making your lunch the prior night, cooking in clump, or precooking all your nourishment and assigning it out for the week in snatch and-go compartments.

The magnificence of meal prep is that it can adjust to accommodate your cooking mastery, lifestyle and individual dietary needs — and it positively doesn't have to resemble a cunningly plated Pinterest-or Instagram-commendable perfect work of art if your aptitudes aren't deserving of a Michelin star.

"Meal prep resembles making your own one of a kind line of microwaveable meals customized to your definite inclinations," says Gabrielle Fundaro, Ph.D., practice science educator, certified game nutritionist and Renaissance Periodization mentor. "Numerous individuals like to pack every one of their morning meals for occupied mornings or snacks to eat at the workplace. Or on the other hand you can likewise pick which meals you'd prefer to prep if you would prefer not to take on each meal for the week."

There are numerous reasons why meal prep is viewed as a best practice for those genuine about arriving at their objectives. Emmie Satrazemis, RD, CSSD, sustenance chief at Trifecta, names the accompanying seven advantages:

1. Allurement Removal.

Ever been hit with hunger and have nothing available to eat? Definitely, that presumably occurs on the every day. Also, maybe the main thing close by is cheap food or that extra birthday cake your associate brought into the workplace. Meal prepping guarantees you generally have choices that fit your dietary needs because you've arranged ahead of time and brought your own nourishment (or have something simple to get from the cooler if you get an instance of the munchies while sitting in front of the TV). This makes adhering to your eating regimen significantly simpler.

2. Absolute Control.

When you are preparing your very own meals or arranging what to eat ahead of time, you get the opportunity to be a complete control crack (positively). You increase total calorie control and large scale parity, and you limit use of undesirable fixings like included sugar, salt and fats. You are likewise guaranteeing you get the best-quality choices and all the more new fixings because you are choosing them yourself.

3. Appetite Manager.

Meal prepping additionally causes you oversee hunger because you can eat when you feel hungry as opposed to holding on to choose and afterward discover a nourishment source. Overseeing hunger often implies you won't gorge when you at long last plunk down for a meal because you won't be as madly hungry.

4. Timesaver.

When done appropriately, meal prepping can spare a lot of time. Regardless of whether you basically pre-hack fixings or cook every one of your meals for the week every Sunday evening, when you return home following a monotonous day, you'll be appreciative you don't need to set aside the effort to go to the store or maybe even cook. This may leave you with more opportunity to work out, play with your children or even appreciate a faultless air pocket shower because you merit it.

5. Cash Saver.

Valuing out your nourishment ahead of time is another bit of the meal-prep condition, which implies your part control currently has cost control. You are likely setting aside cash because you aren't requesting out each lunch and additionally supper and can pick your meal-prep plans dependent on deals at the supermarket if you wish.

6. Squander Eliminator.

This goes connected at the hip with setting aside cash: Once you have a meal-prep routine set up, you'll know precisely the amount of every fixing you need, which likewise eliminates nourishment squander. You'll never again need to observe your products of the soil shrink away in the crisper cabinet while you call for takeout.

7. Stress Remover.

Have you at any point seen how slimming down, particularly cutting calories, can make you consider nourishment all.day.long.? Also, your self-control gets depleted a lot quicker and you are bound to go off your arrangement when no doubt about it "not in the state of mind" to settle on healthier decisions. Meal prepping can help decrease the pressure that accompanies attempting to eat healthier. Fathoming all your nourishment choices ahead of time truly opens up a portion of your self-discipline and mental pressure, helping you arrive at your objectives quicker and without any difficulty.

When it comes to weight loss, the vast majority know the advantages of meal prep: preparing at home causes you control what you eat and deal with your bits. Those are two of the most ideal approaches to shed pounds.

Nonetheless, individuals with the best healthy-gobbling expectations are much of the time entangled when they attempt to put those basic leadership standards enthusiastically without an arrangement.

"When life does precisely what life does-you know, tosses something startling in your way, presents enticing treats that aren't in your arrangement, dangles an unconstrained working environment party time before you-it's anything but difficult to stray away from your best aims," says Kristen Wilk, M.S., R.D.N. "That is, except if you've prepped meals and snacks early."

Wilk says meal-prepping for weight loss-that is, making meals ahead in clumps for your week-is the key for meeting your objectives and healthy-eating desires.

"Having a healthy supper hanging tight for you in your ice chest makes it far simpler to pass on the mozzarella sticks and hot wings at party time," she says. "Realizing you invested energy prepping supplement pressed fixings makes snatching takeout far less alluring."

Here, eight different ways meal prep assists individuals with eating better for weight loss and other healthy objectives.

When you've had a difficult day or have been stuck in an extensive gathering, it's anything but difficult to persuade yourself you should simply run down the road and get a quesadilla or request in a bowl of macintosh and cheddar. Be that as it may, if you have a healthy meal sitting tight for you in the ice chest, you can vanquish the enticement. Your instant meal is nearer and quicker.

"Meal prep takes the mystery and conceivably terrible choices out of nourishment," says Monica Auslander Moreno, M.S., RDN, LDN, originator of Essence Nutrition in Miami. "When you're ravenous at 12:30 p.m., you'll arrange or eat the main thing that crosses your plate. Having a prepped meal decreases nourishment nervousness and instability, and guarantees legitimate nourishment choices."

A prepared to-eat meal additionally makes the hold up in a take-out line or at the drive-through less engaging.

"Picking your meal early additionally evacuates the component of motivation acquiring," says Kelsey Peoples, M.S., RDN, proprietor of The Peoples Plate in New Jersey. "Regardless of whether you're having an especially upsetting day at work, you won't be enticed to snatch a cheeseburger with fries if you as of now have your meal prepared to eat. Research underpins this idea that individuals have generally healthier meals when they preselect their nourishment ahead of time."

You can control what you eat

It's an obvious fact that eatery nourishment, much healthier alternatives like those from popular quick easygoing cafés, simply isn't as healthy as cooking at home. Café meals are reliably higher in sodium and calories. If you eat out for a long time, the additional items can truly include.

With meal prepping, you can gauge and quantify your bits. This can assist you with watching precisely what you're eating, and that makes following calories or different supplements simpler. Additionally, you control the fixings and can ensure your calories are originating from generally supplement thick entire nourishments.

"Eating out will in general incorporate higher-sodium, higher-fat and more fatty dishes because of the fixings, plans and sauces that nourishment administration foundations every now and again use," Wilk says. "It's likewise realized that larger than average segments have become the standard at cafés. By cooking at home, you can serve yourself all the more sensibly."

You can fight off morning hunger

Meal-prepping isn't only for lunch or supper. It can have an enormous effect for individuals who have occupied mornings, as well.

"Medium-term oats are an amazing breakfast that can be prepared the prior night," says Kelly Krikhely, M.S., RD, CDN. "You just blend oats in with Greek yogurt and almond drain or any milk of your decision, and store it in the refrigerator medium-term."

The following morning, you can include nuts, nut spread or organic product to support the nourishment esteem and include enhance.

"If you prep medium-term oats the prior night, you have a filling healthy breakfast you can eat on the run as opposed to snatching the croissant with eggs, bacon and cheddar, or the sugar-loaded biscuit you're accustomed to getting from the corner shop," Krikhely says.

You can remove takeout lunch

Meal prep makes taking lunch to work or school simple and engaging. You don't need to stress over rising right on time to cleave or blend, spread or cut your day's lunch before you leave. Premade meals can be put away in singular get and-go holders and are all set when you are.

"Meal-prepping causes you stay away from the enticements of takeout nourishments, 'prepared to eat' or 'snatch and go' food sources or handled food sources," says Lisa Garcia, M.S., RDN, LD. "These can incorporate a bigger number of calories than you might need to eat and fixings you might need to constrain or maintain a strategic distance from."

Garcia includes, "Rather than spending noon remaining in line at an assume out position, you could take a walk."

Meal prep improves assortment

Research shows that eating an assortment of foods grown from the ground each day can lessen your danger of constant maladies and assist you with bettering deal with your weight.

When you have the opportunity to plan, shop and cook ahead of time, you can be progressively purposeful about what you put on your plate. That implies you can account for a greater amount of those vegetables, natural products, entire grains and healthy fats.

"We generally hear-and state, as health specialists that eating an assortment of nourishments is significant. That is because when you switch up the foods grown from the ground that you're eating, the grains that you cook, or the proteins that you buy, you're likely getting a wide assortment of nutrients and minerals," says Brierley E. Horton, M.S., RD. "So if you set up together a week by week meal plan that is changed in healthy nourishment decisions, you ought to get a decent blend of supplements."

You can modify meals to your needs

Regardless of whether you're attempting to get thinner so you feel much improved, or you have to get in shape because of an ongoing health analysis, meal-prepping can assist you with coordinating your eating regimen objectives something that is extremely difficult to do with eatery nourishment.

"You can alter your meals and snacks to your preferences, inclinations and vitality needs," Wilk says. If you live in a family unit where individuals are following more than one eating routine think a Paleo-eater and a veggie lover cohabitating-meal prep makes it feasible to get two different meals to the table on occupied evenings and mornings. If you prep cauliflower rice and quinoa ahead with a blend of veggies, sauces and proteins, everybody can construct their very own dishes and meals to appreciate. If nothing is prepped ahead of time, eating on the table, not to mention making modified meals, can feel like an unthinkable undertaking.

Meal prep evacuates the pressure of cooking

Following an upsetting day at work, the exact opposite thing you need is to stress over how you'll prepare supper when you don't have a clue what you have in the ice chest. That is the reason numerous individuals go to inexpensive food or takeout. That is one less thing you have on your daily agenda.

Evacuate those stresses by mass cooking on the ends of the week or one day out of every week. This will wipe out the post-work stress and assurance you won't be enticed by the snatch and-go choices at the corner store.

"If you're not a meal organizer as of now, it may feel like a great deal to begin all that time arranging what you'll eat for a week and afterward shopping and prepping," Horton says. "Yet, if you were to include the time gone through consistently considering what's for supper, and afterward making numerous market trips every week, I wager doing it across the board singular motion and before the week gets occupied is going to spare your anxiety."

If the primary week is extreme or confounding, continue onward. "The more you utilize that meal-arranging muscle, the simpler it gets," Horton includes. You can eat cleaner meals

Premade nourishments are often loaded up with additives, salt and different fixings you wouldn't really need to eat if you had the decision. Meal prep gives you that decision.

"When you meal prep, you unavoidably eat 'cleaner,'" Wilk says. That is because you can control what you put on the plate and into your body. Entire nourishments like lean protein, grains, and products of the soil are among the healthiest-and cleanest-food sources you can eat. Meal-prepping makes eating those helpful.

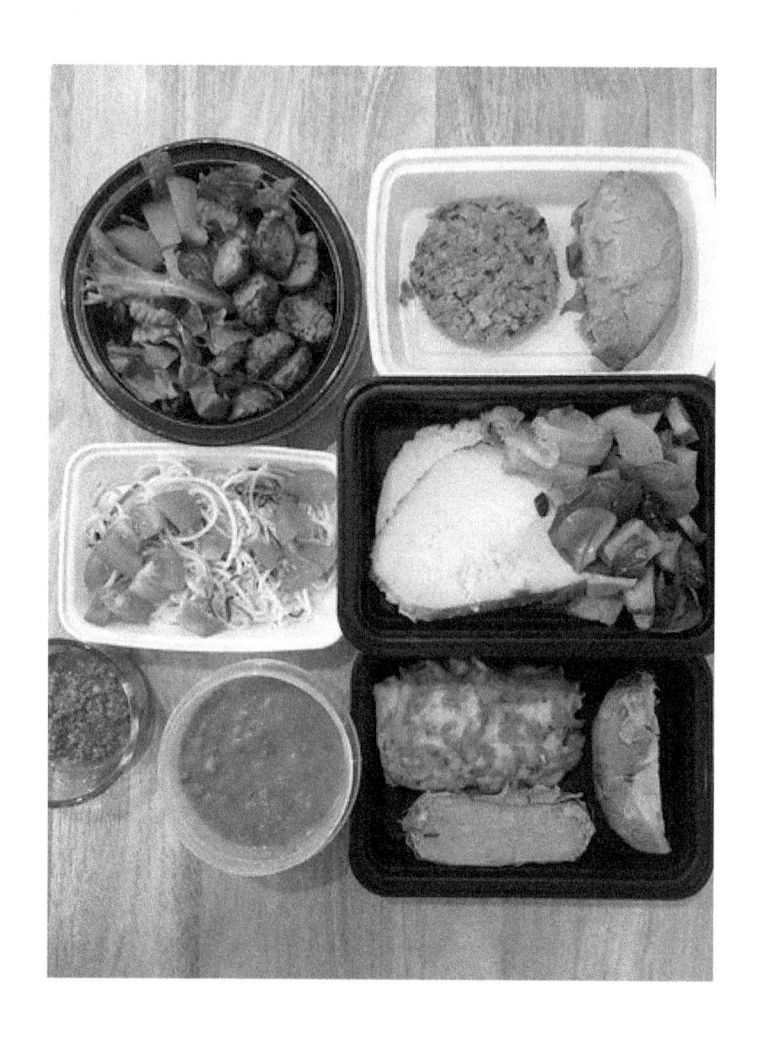

Four Keys to Successful Meal Prep

Regardless of whether you're a first-time meal-prepper or an accomplished one hoping to make the procedure simpler following a while of cooking ahead, these four hints from meal-arranging specialists can assist you with appreciating the movement more and settle on better choices.

1. Start with an ace rundown

"Take a couple of moments to plunk down and work out every one of the meals you regularly cook and your family appreciates," says Amanda Nighbert, M.S., RD. "Having this ace rundown will make arranging your week after week menu so a lot snappier and simpler every week."

Nighbert proposes you should then check what you have close by, in the ice chest, cooler and wash room, and utilize those fixings to finish your decisions for the week. Your lord rundown will assist you with reviewing family-most loved plans, and afterward you can include plans that can assist you with spending fixings and set aside cash when you have to explore new territory.

2. Put aside daily to cook

"Perhaps the greatest boundary I get notification from customers is that they are excessively worn out at night to wash and cut vegetables in the wake of a difficult day at work," Krikhely says. "Many need to eat healthier, however find that preparing supper without any preparation is often a barrier."

Prepping ahead, in any case, encourages you meet and beat that boundary.

"A successful meal-prepper does a lump of the work at once," Nighbert says. "For instance, when I come back from the store every Sunday, I start my meal prep. I go through one to two hours in the kitchen cleaving and cooking as much as I can early to decrease the measure of time to get a meal on the table every night."

3. Start little

If meal-prepping for seven days feels overwhelming, don't consider seven days. Concentrate on three or four. Thusly, you still just need to cook twice in seven days, few out of every odd single day.

"Start with only prepping for a few days or meals," Garcia says. "Beginners particularly can get so centered around 'meal arranging' that they get overpowered and never get the opportunity to do the real prepping. By considering just a few days rather than seven, you're figuring out how to stroll before you attempt to run."

4. Rehash

You don't need to rehash an already solved problem consistently. Rather, get into a cycle of making arrangements for seven days of meals and rehashing it later.

"Spare your week after week meal plans for a couple of months so you can return and reuse a whole week's arrangement on ends of the week when you're lacking in time," Horton proposes.

A HELPFUL HEALTHY EATING STRATEGY

Who hasn't gone home late with a snarling stomach however little vitality to shop and cook? A bustling timetable is one of the top reasons why individuals pick fast takeout meals, which are often calorie-loaded and a supporter of growing waistlines. [1-3]

Presently, envision a different situation where inside a couple of moments of strolling through the entryway you have a scrumptious home-prepared supper, and maybe even lunch pressed up for the following day. In the midst of furious weekday plans, meal prep or meal arranging is an incredible device to help keep us on a healthy eating track. Albeit any sort of meal prep requires arranging, there is nobody right strategy, as it can differ dependent on nourishment inclinations, cooking capacity, timetables, and individual objectives. Here are a few models:

If you currently eat cheap food or takeout a few evenings of the week, your objective might be to pick a specific day of the week to make a nourishment shopping rundown and hit the market.

If you as of now nourishment shop once every week and have essential cooking abilities, your objective might be to pick one day seven days to do the greater part of the cooking, or attempt another formula.

If you as of now cook some weekday meals for your family, you may choose to make a timetable with the goal that you are not choosing a minute ago what to make and to guarantee you have the required fixings close by.

A few advantages of meal prep:

Can help set aside cash

Can eventually spare time

Can help with weight control, as you choose the fixings and bits served

Can add to a general all the more healthfully adjusted eating routine

Can diminish worry as you evade a minute ago choices about what to eat, or hurried preparation

Prepping for Meal Prep

Talk about with your family what kinds of nourishments and most loved meals they like to eat.

Start a month to month schedule or spreadsheet to record your meal thoughts, most loved formula destinations, and nourishment shopping records.

Gather healthy plans. Clasp plans from print magazines and papers and spare in a fastener, or duplicate connections of plans onto an online spreadsheet.

Think about specific meals or nourishments for different days of the week. Recollect Wednesday as Prince Spaghetti Day? A few families appreciate the consistency of comprehending what's in store, and it can facilitate your meal arranging. Models are Meatless Mondays, Whole Grain Wednesdays, Stir-Fry Fridays, and so forth.

Start little: Aim to make enough suppers for 2-3 days of the week.

Beginning

Case of a meal preparation calendarChoose a specific day of the week to: 1) plan the menu, regardless of whether step by step or for the entire month, and work out your basic food item list 2) nourishment shop, 3) do meal prep, or the majority of your cooking. A portion of nowadays may cover if you pick, yet separating these undertakings may help keep meal arranging sensible.

As you discover top pick 'prep-capable' meals, or your menus become progressively well-known and steady, watch for deals and coupons to load up on oftentimes utilized rack stable fixings like pasta, rice, and other entire grains, lentils, beans (canned or dried), jostled sauces, healthy oils, and flavors.

On your meal prep day, center first around nourishments that take the longest to cook: proteins like chicken and fish; entire grains like dark colored rice, quinoa, and farro; dried beans and vegetables; and, broiled vegetables.

Additionally consider preparing staple nourishments that everybody in the family appreciates and which you can without much of a stretch add to a weekday meal or get for a tidbit: washed greens for a serving of mixed greens, hardboiled eggs, a bowl of slashed organic product, cooked beans.

If you lean toward not to pre-cook proteins, consider marinating poultry, fish, or even tofu on your prep day with the goal that you can rapidly pop them into the stove or sautéed food later in the week.

Perform multiple tasks! While nourishments are preparing or rising on the stovetop, slash vegetables and crisp natural product, or wash and dry serving of mixed greens for later in the week.

When you cook a formula, make additional parts for one more day or two of meals, or to solidify for a different week. Make certain to date and name what goes in the cooler so you recognize what you have close by.

For snacks, get a head-begin and utilize singular meal compartments. Separation prepared nourishment into the holders on prep day.

Capacity

Meal prep can set aside time and cash if you are preparing only enough for what is required the next week. Refrigeration and solidifying are a significant advance to effective meal arranging. Nonetheless, overlooked nourishment, for example, produce covering up in a cabinet or a stew put away on a back rack in a hazy compartment for a really long time can ruin and prompt nourishment squander. Mark all prepped things with a date so you can follow when to utilize them by. Turn put away things with the goal that the most seasoned nourishments/meals are kept in advance. Store profoundly transitory things like greens, herbs, and hacked organic products up front at eye-level so you make sure to utilize them.

When it comes to solidifying, a few nourishments work superior to other people. Prepared meals will in general stop well in hermetically sealed compartments. Nourishments with high dampness content, for example, plate of mixed greens, tomatoes, or watermelon, are not prescribed as they will in general become soft when solidified and defrosted. Whitening vegetables for a couple of moments before solidifying can help. In any case, if the surface of a solidified nourishment gets unfortunate in the wake of defrosting, they may even now be utilized in cooked plans, for example, soups and stews.

Coming up next are prescribed occasions for different cooked nourishments that offer the best flavors, most extreme supplements, and sanitation.

Refrigeration at 40°F or lower

1-2 days: Cooked ground poultry or ground meat

3-4 days: Cooked entire meats, fish and poultry; soups and stews

5 days: Cooked beans; hummus multi week: Hard bubbled eggs; hacked vegetables if put away in hermetically sealed compartment

2 weeks: Soft cheddar, opened

5 a month and a half: Hard cheddar, opened

Solidifying at 0°F or lower

2-3 months: Soups and stews; cooked beans

3-6 months: Cooked or ground meat and poultry

6-8 months: Berries and hacked organic product (banana, apples, pears, plums, mango) put away in a cooler sack

8 a year: Vegetables, if whitened first for around 3-5 minutes (contingent upon the vegetable)

Prepared to begin? The following are a few plans that loan well to greater groups—and remember that the Healthy Eating Plate can fill in as an accommodating menu arranging guide. Glad prepping!

Farro with Confetti Vegetables

Veggie lover Shepherd's Pie

Cauliflower Tomato Soup with Indian Spices

Stirred Up Grains

White Beans, Wild Rice, and Mushrooms

Vegetable Stock (incredible for utilizing remaining veggie trimmings)

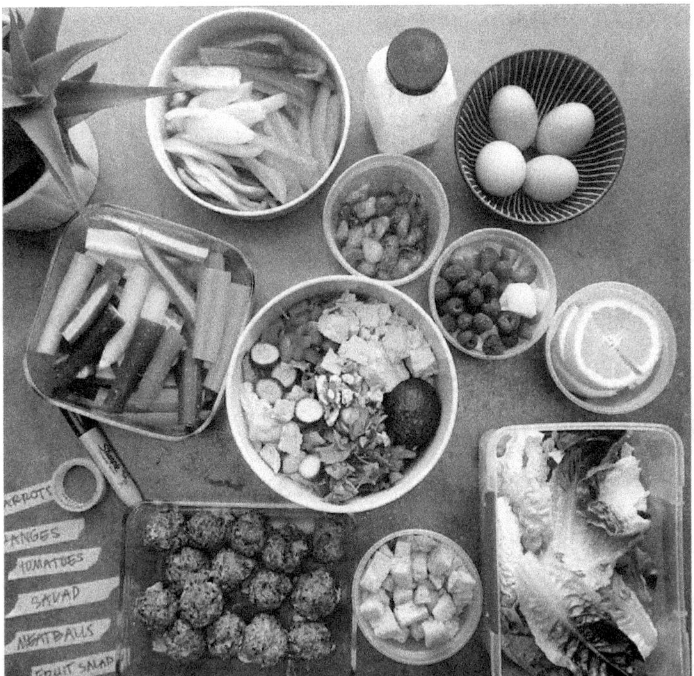
ARROTS
ANGES
TOMATOES
SALAD
MEATBALLS
FRUIT SALAD

STEP BY STEP TIPS TO START A MEAL PREP

1. Make a revolution with your preferred modest meal prep plans

One of the keys to meal prepping is to keep things as straightforward as could be expected under the circumstances. Nowadays, I adhere to a short rundown of modest meal prep plans (like these moderate cooker carnitas) that I pivot through on a month to month premise. This removes the mystery from meal arranging each week.

2. Discover Ingredient Overlaps

This is perhaps the best thing you can do to have a simple meal prep. My preferred thing is to make 3-4 lbs of meat and afterward discover approaches to join it into different meals. It makes my meal prep simpler and less expensive because I don't need to purchase the same number of fixings This likewise gives you not too bad assortment consistently.

3. Cleave veggies early

The greatest time-suck in meal prepping is cleaving vegetables, particularly onions! They make me cry EVERY SINGLE TIME. I can't resist. Yet, I cracking adoration onions, so I push through the torment. The point however, is that hacking vegetables each meal is a tremendous time channel. If you would prefer not to really prep an entire meal, one basic hint is to simply prep your vegetables at an opportune time in the week.

4. Break out the slow cooker

The #1 approach to have a simple meal prep is to utilize a slow cooker! Dump the fixings in, turn it on, and hold up 6-8 hours. There truly is no simpler method to make seven days of meals early.

5. Get the best meal prep compartments

If you truly need your meal prepping to be as simple as would be prudent, then you need to put resources into these meal prep holders. Crystal makes putting away, warming, and cleaning 10x simpler.

6. You don't need to cook all that you prep

I like to eat a large portion of my vegetables newly cooked instead of following 3-4 days in the ice chest, so whenever my wife and I finish our week by week staple outing, I as a rule go through an hour tuning in to a web recording while I cleave up and sack seven days of vegetables. The less work I need to do to eat healthy, the better.

7. Start Small and Simple

If you're new to meal prepping, don't attempt to make and prepare a whole week of nourishment on your first endeavor! Set aside some effort to realize what plans you love and start little. You would prefer not to burn through a lot of time and cash on a meal you won't appreciate. These medium-term oats plans are overly simple to make and begin with!

8. Put it in your timetable

"Inability to design is wanting to fizzle."

I abhor that statement because it's so cracking mushy. But on the other hand it's valid. If you never plan to meal prep, then you never will. Put aside a period in your week by week schedule and close it off for meal prep.

9. Utilize a meal organizer

I've been meal prepping for such a long time that it's generally instinctive for me. If you're new to meal prepping, then go get an organizer like this one! You can outline your week after week meal plan, plans, basic food item list, and so on.

10. Very much loaded ice chest/cooler/wash room

There's nothing more baffling than not having that one fixing that you have to finish a meal! We do whatever it takes not to purchase more than we need, however we do have a rundown of staples that we keep available. We generally have a pack of chicken (2-3lbs) and our preferred flavors close by so that if we're after all other options have been exhausted we can make some flame broiled chicken for the week!

11. Prepare fixings early

You don't need to do a monstrous meal prep without fail. Here and there prepping a couple of fixings can go far to sparing you time consistently. I'll cut up carrots, cucumbers, chime peppers and have some all set veggie snacks consistently!

Techniques To Meal Prep On A Budget

1. If you're evaluating another formula, adhere to the normal sum.

After you've tried it out, don't hesitate to twofold or triple the sum so you can have increasingly remaining. The exact opposite thing you need to do is go through a lot of cash just to prepare a meal you don't care for by any means.

2. Purchase in Bulk

The most straightforward approach to meal prep on a spending limit is to purchase however much nourishment in mass as could be expected. You can get meat, rice, potatoes, oats and a wide range of flavors and canned merchandise in mass. Purchasing in mass possibly bodes well if you realize you'll eat it before everything turns sour.

I eat a huge amount of protein and one of my preferred approaches to stack up on meat is when markets run deals. Walmart, HEB, and some different stores do this, however when nourishment is near lapsing, they'll mark it route down. This is an extraordinary time to stock up and stick it in the cooler.

3. Unit Price per Food

If you're attempting to meal prep on a spending limit, the most significant thing is to watch out for the unit cost for the nourishment you're purchasing. The less you pay per ounce or pound of nourishment, the better.

4. Eat Less Meat

If you're utilized to a high protein diet, then you realize how costly meat can be. If you can discover approaches to eat sub in less expensive protein sources like nuts, beans, or dairy items, it tends to be an immense cash saver. Eating less meat is by a wide margin the simplest method to prep modest meals.

5. Decrease Food Waste

The normal American discards over $600 per year in nourishment! Probably the most effortless approaches to meal prep on a financial limit is to just eat the nourishment you purchase. The less nourishment you discard, the less nourishment you need to purchase!

6. Meal plan dependent on what's at a bargain

A great many people get to the store, purchase everything on their rundown, and afterward want to discover a few coupons en route. Probably the most ideal approaches to meal prep on a financial limit is to design your meals dependent on what is at a bargain at the store. This will help you truly make some modest meals and spend less on staple goods.

7. Stop it

Whenever I make bean stew or soup, I attempt to make enough to solidify for the days where we haven't had the opportunity to pass by the store and don't have any nourishment. The greatest shortcoming when it comes to eating out is the craving for accommodation. I'm tied in with finding simple meal prep plans! If you have any top choices, share them in the remarks beneath!

8. Get out the storeroom and cooler

Go investigate your storeroom and cooler! It's unreasonably simple for storeroom and cooler nourishments to fire heaping up. You most likely have a lot of half-eaten packs of rice, oats, corn meal, and pasta.

If you're hoping to spare a touch of money the following hardly any months then do a brisk mind all that you have loaded up to and utilize those nourishments for your next meal prep.

9. Keep comfort meals close by

The greatest eating regimen and spending executioner is comfort. In the wake of a monotonous day at work it is too simple to even think about stopping by chipotle in transit home. Having out for lunch and those snappy take-out stops can rapidly include and break your spending limit.

Having a couple of accommodation meals close by can go far towards remaining steady. We love to make bean stew and stop half so we generally have a meal prepared to warm up after all other options have been exhausted.

10. Shop at less expensive stores

A simple method to meal prep on a spending limit is to shop at less expensive stores. Spots like costco, walmart, and ALDI will in general be less expensive than upper-scale markets like Trader Joe's and Whole Foods.

11. Eat nourishment in-season

Products of the soil are staples of any eating regimen, however they can have wide swings in cost contingent upon the season. Here and there we'll see blueberries and strawberries going for $1/lb and different occasions they'll be 3-4x as costly!

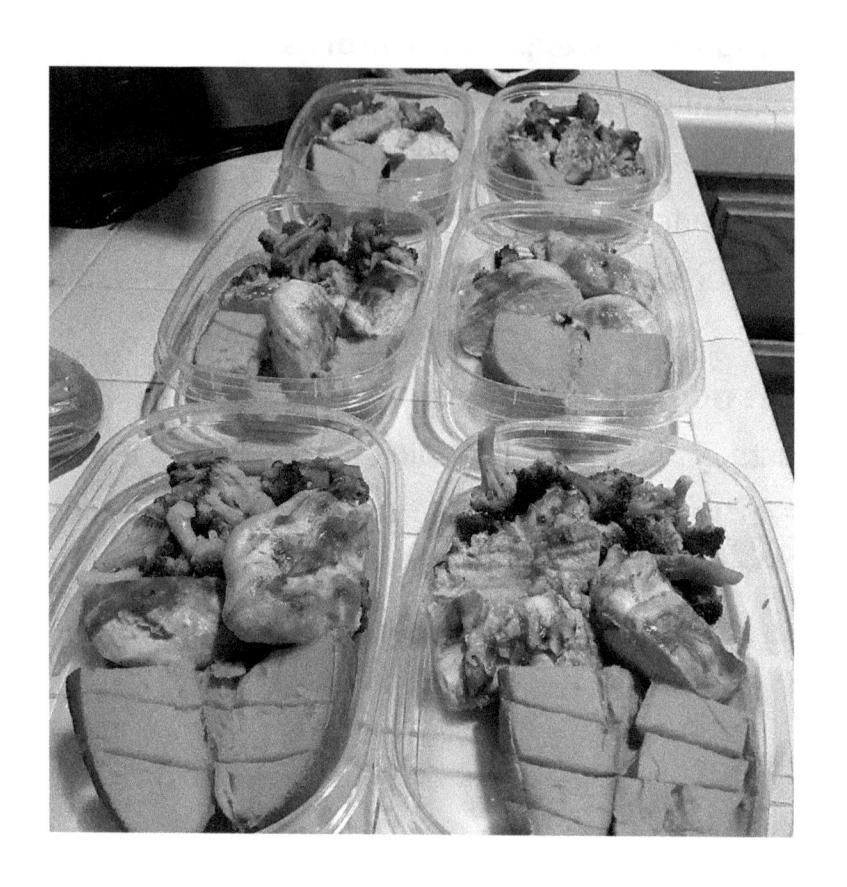

EXTREME GRAB-AND-GO BREAKFASTS YOU CAN MEAL-PREP

Lift your hand if breakfast implies bringing down a bowl of oat before hurrying out the entryway. Or on the other hand a donut off that plate in your office's regular room. Or on the other hand even only a hurriedly gulped mug of espresso at your work area.

That is correct, we feel your sugar crash and caffeine surge.

Despite the fact that less individuals are having breakfast by any stretch of the imagination, it's as yet considered the "most significant" meal of the day. A few examinations show that having a well-adjusted breakfast has benefits for physical and mental health.

But on the other hand the meal the vast majority of us don't possess energy for. That is the place meal-prepping proves to be useful — to ensure you have great, healthy eats close by each morning.

We're taking make-ahead breakfast plans above and beyond with this gathering and offering you 17 meals that are anything but difficult to make ahead and convenient.

Lift your hand if breakfast implies bringing down a bowl of grain before hurrying out the entryway. Or on the other hand a donut off that plate in your office's basic room. Or on the other hand even only a quickly gulped mug of espresso at your work area.

Correct, we feel your sugar crash and caffeine surge.

Despite the fact that less individuals are having breakfast by any means, it's as yet considered the "most significant" meal of the day. A few investigations show that having a well-adjusted breakfast has benefits for physical and mental health. But at the same time the meal the greater part of us don't possess energy for. That is the place meal-prepping proves to be useful — to ensure you have great, healthy eats close by each morning.

We're taking make-ahead breakfast plans above and beyond with this gathering and offering you 17 meals that are anything but difficult to make ahead and versatile.

So hit that nap button once again. You can snatch something healthy from your very own kitchen and go.

Make-Ahead Breakfast Bowls are loaded with filling, healthy fixings to control you through your morning. This veggie lover and without gluten breakfast formula is likewise cooler agreeable!

Get going, it's morning meal time!

Half a month back I referenced I've been attempting to have a legitimate breakfast every morning and it's been doing some incredible things for my vitality levels. A filling meal with protein, fat, and sugars first thing in the ay em totally establishes the pace for a gainful day, and if I skip breakfast it feels as if there's a 10 pound weight on my head. Like a cover of haze is blurring my vision and my face gauges like, 100 pounds. If you don't mind reveal to me you can relate?

Peculiar facial issues aside, let's face it, making breakfast a need is unbelievably difficult in the mornings. Unavoidably the dishwasher should be exhausted, Lincoln's school nibble needs pressed and he obviously needs a healthy breakfast, preparing espresso is an absolute necessity, lastly it's nutrients for all. After a short time it's an ideal opportunity to stack up the vehicle and head out to class, or hurry up to my office for the afternoon. In light of what has been said, speedy and simple morning meals are the name of the game recently and these Breakfast Bowls are killing it in the scrumptious division, yet they're make ahead (warm in ONE moment!) and cooler inviting as well.

Make-Ahead-Breakfast-Bowls-Freezer-Friendly-iowagirleats-02

Have you at any point heard the maxim "have breakfast like a ruler, lunch like a sovereign, and supper like a poor person"? I'm burrowing it. All things considered, typically breakfast and supper are both eaten like I'm the Queen of England, however to me a healthy breakfast has a major effect in how my day goes.

Make-Ahead Breakfast Bowls contain a generous mix of custom made Potatoes o' Brien (potatoes with green pepper and onion, you all, which smell UNBELIEVABLE while cooking!) plush fried eggs, newly destroyed cheddar, and hot green onions which are commended by my preferred egg blending – tortilla chips and salsa – then presented hot and crisp, or divvied up into individual measured compartments to store in the icebox or cooler to snatch, warm, and go, throughout the entire week. I've been making a cluster of Breakfast Bowls on Sundays then warming in the microwave during insane weekday mornings. They're super filling and, while I do love a morning meal of berries, a banana, and hand crafted pecan margarine, I'll scarcely ever turn down something sweltering and generous – particularly in this climate!

I made these dishes to be vegan, yet if you'd like somewhat more protein, feel free to darker up 3/4lb breakfast hotdog or bacon and add them to the dishes. Dice or concoction new avocado to include increasingly healthy and fulfilling fats to the bowl, or potentially catch a tortilla and make your own morning meal burrito with the fixings. Presently go forward, and easily devour breakfast – as it's been said, clear eyes, full stomach, can't lose! (Or something to that effect...)

Start by slashing 2lb Yukon Gold potatoes, 1 green ringer pepper, and 1 enormous onion into 1" 3D shapes then adding them to a huge sheet container.

Shower the vegetables with additional virgin olive oil then sprinkle on a liberal measure of natively constructed prepared salt, and pepper. Hurl with your hands to equitably cover the vegetables, then move half to another sheet dish. This guarantees there's sufficient space for the vegetables to cook and get pleasant and caramelized versus steaming from being packed together on one sheet skillet.

Broil the two searches for gold 40 minutes, or until the potatoes are brilliant darker and delicate, blending the vegetables and turning the skillet partially through.

Psst: If you're fixing your dish with foil, make certain to shower them with nonstick splash first – it truly has any kind of effect!

In the interim, whisk 12 enormous eggs with salt and pepper in a huge bowl.

Splash an enormous skillet over medium warmth with nonstick shower then include the eggs and scramble until they're scarcely cooked through – they should at present be somewhat smooth and glossy.

Last stop – gathering! Heap the potatoes and eggs into bowls then top with newly destroyed cheddar and slashed green onions. Like I stated, I love eggs with tortilla chips and salsa, so I tucked those into my morning meal bowls before eating as well. A diced avocado or guacamole would be Heavenly also!

Make-Ahead Breakfast Bowls

Fixings

SERVES 6

2lbs yukon gold potatoes, hacked into 1" blocks

1 green pepper, seeded then hacked into 1" blocks

1 onion, hacked into 1" blocks additional virgin olive oil hand crafted sans gluten prepared salt (see notes for formula) and pepper

12 eggs

4oz newly destroyed cheddar

3 green onions, hacked

Fixings: avocado, tortilla chips, salsa

6 individual-sized tupperware or glass compartments with tops

Headings

Preheat broiler to 425 degrees. Include potatoes, peppers, and onions to a huge sheet skillet then shower with additional virgin olive oil, natively constructed prepared salt, and pepper and afterward hurl until equitably covered. Move a large portion of the vegetables to a subsequent sheet container then dish the two prospects 40 minutes, or until potatoes are brilliant darker and delicate, blending and turning skillet part of the way through.

In the meantime, split eggs into an enormous bowl then season with salt and pepper and speed until smooth. Warmth a huge skillet over medium warmth then splash with nonstick shower and include eggs. Scramble until the eggs are scarcely cooked through and still marginally glossy then scoop onto a plate and put in a safe spot.

Partition the potatoes and eggs equitably between the holders then put aside to cool. When cool, sprinkle with cheddar and green onions then cover and refrigerate. Stop any bits that aren't eaten inside three days.

To warm from solidified: microwave at half power for 1-1/2 minutes then mix and keep microwaving until nourishment is warmed, blending between interims. Top with discretionary fixings then serve.

Presently, the excellence of these make-ahead breakfast bowls is that they're flawless to keep in the cooler and cooler for snappy and generous morning meals throughout the entire week. You'll should simply partition the eggs and potatoes between six cooler agreeable compartments then enable them to cool somewhat. Top with destroyed cheddar and green onions then snap a top on top. Store in the ice chest for as long as three days, or reserve in the cooler for 1-2 months.

To warm from the cooler, microwave the dishes on half power for 1-1/2 minutes, mix, and afterward microwave on full power until warmed through, mixing like clockwork or thereabouts.

Regardless of whether you have these Make-Ahead Breakfast Bowls immediately, or warm every morning, appreciate long stretches of vitality ahead!

AVOCADO AND EGG BREAKFAST MEAL PREP

Put your meal-prep compartments to great use with these generous breakfast bowls. With darker rice, sautéed kale, avocado, and hard-bubbled egg, this well-adjusted breakfast is healthy enough to shield your stomach from snarling midmorning.

Energizing your body and brain is fundamental to adapt to the bustling day ahead. The correct nourishments assist you with centering rationally and stay stimulated physically.

What's more, this specific breakfast bowl is so easy to make.

The eggs can be prepared just as you would prefer. My top choice (and generally healthy) are poached eggs. Eggs give a huge amount of extraordinary supplements and protein.

The dark colored rice can be prepared in an enormous cluster prepared for the week preceding breakfast. Darker rice gives your great carbs and fiber. These carbs will keep your vitality up for the duration of the day.

The kale gives a portion of day by day greens and nutrients. Sautéing the kale with garlic and discretionary red pepper drops offers it a stunning enhancing which praises the eggs and rice. You can likewise swap out the kale for simmered brussels grows, butternut squash or peas.

The avocado gives you your great fats which can help bring down the awful cholesterol in your body and help your skin and hair.

Sounds like a triumphant breakfast to me – stimulated with incredible skin and hair!

Fixings:

1/2 cup darker rice

6 enormous eggs

2 tablespoons olive oil

2 cloves garlic, minced

1/4 teaspoon squashed red pepper drops, discretionary

4 cups slashed kale

1/4 cup naturally ground Parmesan

1 avocado, divided, seeded, stripped and cut

Headings:

In an enormous pot of 1 cup water, cook rice as indicated by bundle directions; put in a safe spot.

Spot eggs in a huge pan and spread with cold water by 1 inch. Heat to the point of boiling and cook for 1 moment. Spread eggs with a tight-fitting cover and expel from heat; put in a safe spot for 8-10 minutes. Channel well and let cool before stripping and splitting. Warmth olive oil in a huge skillet over medium high warmth. Include garlic and red pepper pieces, if utilizing. Cook, blending every now and again, until fragrant, around 1-2 minutes. Mix in kale until shriveled, around 5-6 minutes. Mix in Parmesan.

Spot rice, eggs, kale and avocado into meal prep compartments.

BANANA AND CHOCOLATE CHIP PREPARED OATMEAL CUPS

Try not to pass up an extraordinary wellspring of fiber and heart-healthy oats because you have no opportunity to make it on the stove. Put the blend in a biscuit tin and heat, and you have get and-go oats. Indeed, chocolate chips must be included, clearly.

I have another heated oatmeal cup formula for you. My arrangement was to share this later in the week however I continue getting LOTS of messages requesting the formula so your desire is my direction. I will share this formula today.

This formula was enlivened by a great deal of excessively ready bananas sitting on my counter. I know weighty. The vast majority of them I solidified for smoothies however chose to keep a couple out for because I had the inclination to make a banana formula. From the outset I thought banana bread. Yet, then I thought if I make banana bread we will eat that portion before the day's over and I needed to make something that would last somewhat longer than that. I likewise thought breakfast treats yet again those eventual passed before the day's over. My children can't avoid any treat and in all honesty neither can I. Then my formula light went off. Banana and chocolate chip heated oatmeal! My children love prepared oatmeal however for reasons unknown they realize this is only a morning meal nourishment so they don't breathe in it across the board sitting.

This heated oatmeal formula is delicious! It unquestionably has the kinds of banana bread and a morning meal treat enveloped with a healthy heated oatmeal cup.

If you incline toward video over picture directions then look at this snappy formula instructional exercise I set up together on this banana and chocolate chip heated oatmeal formula.

The chocolate chips are clearly a treat, particularly for breakfast. If you need to forget about them then proceed. Nonetheless, there is just ½ cup in the formula so if you need a little chocolate fix then toss some in. Feel free to toss them in, you will be cheerful you did.

Much the same as my other heated oatmeal cup plans these stop superbly. After they are cooled wrap independently in cling wrap then spot in a huge cooler pack. I warm mine up in the microwave for 2 minutes on high. I suggest warming up close by an espresso cup of water. This little cooler cooking tip will keep the surface of the prepared oatmeal cup delicate and clammy.

The banana and unadulterated maple syrup in the formula includes a decent measure of sweetness. Yet, if you need all the more then pour some additional maple syrup over the top before you eat it.

Each prepared oatmeal cup is 202 calories and 6 weight watchers focuses in addition to.

Fixings

3 cups moved oats or antiquated oats

½ teaspoon ground cinnamon

⅛ teaspoon ground nutmeg

1 teaspoon heating powder

¼ teaspoon salt

2 enormous eggs

¼ cup unadulterated maple syrup

1 cup squashed banana, 2 bananas

2 teaspoons unadulterated vanilla concentrate

1 cup 1% milk

¼ cup dissolved coconut oil

1 cup small chocolate chips

Cooking splash.

Directions

Preheat stove to 350.

In a medium bowl consolidate the moved oats, cinnamon, nutmeg, preparing powder, and salt. Put in a safe spot.

Split the 2 eggs into another medium bowl. Whisk together with the maple syrup, pounded banana, and vanilla concentrate till the fixings are consolidated and smooth.

Gradually race in the milk and coconut oil.

Empty the wet fixings into the dry fixings. Mix until every one of the oats are secured and soaked.

Gradually mix in the chocolate chips.

Shower a biscuit skillet with cooking splash then partition the oatmeal blend among the 12 biscuits tins. Press the blend down with a spoon so every one of the oats are shrouded in fluid.

Heat for 30 minutes or until the tops are marginally dark colored.

Let cool for 5 minutes. Appreciate with a little unadulterated maple syrup.

EGG BISCUITS WITH HAM, KALE, AND CAULIFLOWER RICE

Not an ounce of dairy or a grain in locate in these veggie-pressed biscuits, which get genuinely great flavor from diced ham. Discussion about super-fulfilling. Recollect the Thai eggs benedict and cauliflower misuses? At times he doesn't care for my thoughts.

These are generally the days that I make paleo enchantment treat bars or paleo lemon bars to reestablish our relationship and my "great wife who sustains her significant other ordinary things now and then" status.

You comprehend.

Along these lines, in the mission to accomplish typical formula ness OBVIOUSLY, my reasoning gadget then went to Dr. Seuss. We as a whole realize he is the EPITOME of commonality and general not odd individual age.

That is to say, similar to Mr. Seuss, I ate these green eggs and ham biscuits in a pontoon with a goat, while gliding in a canal, and I am 100% ordinary.

Be that as it may, I may be lying. In any case, just around 1 thing. Is it eating biscuits with a goat OR being ordinary?

This is gaining out of power. Back to ham.

We've eaten a couple of assortments of egg biscuits on here (The Egg Muffins with Maple Sweet Potato Noodles being my most loved and Keto Low Carb Egg Muffins with Ham being next in line) because, well, I am somewhat fixated on simple breakfast meal prep plans and am ALWAYS watchful for healthy meal prep thoughts for the week.

Also, I realize you are as well, because you're beautiful faces continue mentioning them. So BAM! Here you go. It's sort of having a mid-being-composed life emergency.

Whatever that implies.

Not exclusively are these lone 5 INGREDIENTS (whoopee for not including the quantity of fixings with a number cruncher. Possibly.) thus simple that my pooch could most likely make them WITHOUT thumbs, they additionally happen to be sans dairy.

I know, you don't imagine that is a major dealio. In any case, it is..because MR. FFF enjoyed them.

Furthermore, it's the first occasion when I have served him eggs without cheddar that he has enjoyed.

I can't lie. I was stressed over not welcoming ooey-mushy yums into our comfortable, tin-formed gathering. It just GOES with eggs.

Be that as it may, the center o-rama is attempting this new gluten/grain/dairy free diet (so stay tuned for more plans) so I would not like to resemble "Goodness YOU L-O-V-E ham and eggs for breakfast?" OH THESE ARE SO GOOD... .BUT YOU CAN'T EAT THEM."

That would win me about - 8 great wife focuses.

Be that as it may, then we both tasted them. What's more, they were in reality BETTER than without the cheddar that-never-was (??) because the salty, hammy goodness had the option to SHINE through, similar to the protein-start that it is.

They're yummy in your belly, you can eat them WHILE you get down to business AND you can even live in a fantasy world that a celebrated book was expounded on your dietary patterns.

Not while you drive however. If it's not too much trouble focus out and about and utilize that creative mind once you get to the workplace.

Fixings

1 Cup Cauliflower cut into scaled down pieces

3 Large eggs

1 Cup Kale or spinach, daintily pressed and attacked scaled down pieces

3/4 Cup Pasture-raised Ham intensely pressed and cut into scaled down 3D shapes

Salt

Pepper

Directions

Preheat your stove to 400 degrees and liberally shower a]muffin tin with cooking splash. Put in a safe spot.

In a little nourishment processor(mine is 3 cups) process the cauliflower until separated and it takes after rice. Put in a safe spot.

In a huge bowl, whisk the eggs. Include the kale, ham, cauliflower rice and season with a touch of salt and pepper. Blend well.

Gap the blend between 6 biscuit tins* and afterward prepare until the eggs feel set, around 20 minutes.

Give cool access the container and afterward DEVOUR.

THINGS I ALWAYS DO WHEN MEAL PREPPING

Since I've been meal prepping normally for well more than two years, I am persuaded it is probably the best thing you can accomplish for yourself (and your family) to make weekday mealtimes a mess simpler.

While the intricate details of meal prep will fluctuate dependent on your needs, inclinations, and timetable, there are some broad standards that consistently apply. Here are the seven things I generally do when meal prepping.

1. I evaluate my calendar for the coming week.

The sum and kind of nourishment I meal prep changes week to week dependent on a couple of different factors, yet to be specific my timetable. Half a month I have supper at home each night, different weeks I have supper out on more than one occasion, and still others I have consecutive early mornings, which means I need a simple snatch and-go breakfast choice. To endeavor sure my meal prep endeavors coordinate with my needs, it is fundamental to initially evaluate my timetable for the coming week.

2. I close off at any rate 30 minutes.

There is no chance to get around it: Meal prep requires some investment. The careful measure of time relies upon what works best for you. However, I've discovered that the best meal prep sessions require closing off 30 minutes (albeit ideally 60 minutes) with the goal that I can be 100 percent centered around the job needing to be done.

3. I make an arrangement of activity.

I'm sure nothing can make meal prep all the more overpowering, threatening, or baffling than jumping into a prep session without having a strategy. In other words, an arranged rundown (mental or composed) of precisely what I intend to achieve. It is the main thing I do in each meal prep session. It encourages me identify which nourishments take the longest to cook and the fixings I'll require. Furthermore, the greater part of each of the, a strategy keeps me sorted out and limits my time in the kitchen.

4. I pick plans that make great remains.

When it comes to meal prep, not all plans are made equivalent. Since the reason of meal prep is cooking nourishments since you can eat consistently, one of my top markers for picking plans is pondering if they make great remains.

5. I cook different things one after another.

For me, meal prep is tied in with performing multiple tasks. To utilize my time, I generally try to cook various things on the double. For instance, while a plate of chicken thighs are broiling in the broiler, I can stew a pot of quinoa on the stove, and get a pot of hard-bubbled eggs going simultaneously.

6. I haul out capacity compartments early.

There is nothing more awful than completing meal prep just to understand that the capacity holders I need to utilize are now pressed full or are filthy and in the dishwasher. This has happened a bigger number of times than I want to share, however I think I've at last taken in my exercise.

7. I make an arrangement for how to transform my prepped nourishment into meals.

It's a major misuse of your time, cash, and nourishment when you don't really eat the nourishment you put the exertion into prepping. In any event, when I don't have an express meal plan, I generally take a couple of moments after meal prepping to consider (and typically record!) a free arrangement for how I'll exploit such nourishment in the coming week.

THINGS I WISH SOMEONE TOLD ME BEFORE I STARTED MEAL PREPPING

I've been meal prepping for over two years now, and I've discovered that the best exercises I've taken in have originated from tying on my cover, getting in the kitchen, and doing it throughout each and every week. When it comes to meal prep, experience truly is the best educator, and I've discovered my furrow through heaps of experimentation. Thinking back on everything, here are some significant exercises that I've learned en route.

1. Meal prep isn't one-size-fits-all.

There is definitely not a supernatural recipe for meal prep. What works for me probably won't work for you, and the other way around. It very well may be useful to perceive what (and how) others meal prep for motivation, however toward the day's end it's tied in with making sense of a framework that works for youthat addresses your issues.

2. It doesn't need to look the equivalent consistently.

Similarly as different schedules work for different individuals, they can likewise shift from week to week. While a little while it's useful to prepare most meals for the week early, others may include doing only each thing in turn — like making a clump of medium-term oats, marinating chicken, or hacking vegetables. I've figured out how to grasp an evolving plan, because I know my meal prep needs will probably change from week to week.

3. Prep doesn't need to occur on a Sunday, or at the same time.

We often talk about end of the week or Sunday meal prep, however in all actuality, meal prep can happen whenever of the week. The key is finding the day that is least demanding to close off a lump of time — possibly that is Sunday, however perhaps it's Tuesday or Wednesday. What's more, perhaps that day varies from week to week, and that is additionally absolutely OK.

Meghan likewise as of late instructed me that meal prep doesn't really need to happen at the same time. As a mother of two with a bustling calendar, she spreads a couple of short meal prep sessions through the span of a few days.

4. Working out a course of action early can truly help.

For me, this has been a complete distinct advantage for a progressively effective meal prep schedule. What's more, as somebody who cherishes manually written records, I'm shocked I haven't been doing this from the beginning. I start by making a composed, requested rundown of the considerable number of errands I intend to achieve during meal prep. It causes me identify which nourishments take the longest to cook and the fixings I'll require. Also, the greater part of all, having a course of action keeps me sorted out and limits my time in the kitchen.

5. It's justified, despite all the trouble to put resources into great stockpiling holders.

I at last got around to getting some not too bad meal prep stockpiling compartments a month ago, and I truly wish I put resources into them quite a while in the past. Out of a balance of apathy and lingering, I depended on a jumble of old, worn out holders, a significant number of which didn't contain tops.

Regardless of whether you meal prep a little or a great deal, help yourself out and get some great compartments. Extra focuses if they're cooler, microwave-, and broiler safe.

6. You can generally meal prep — regardless of whether you don't meal plan.

When I began meal prepping, it generally went ahead the impact points of meal arranging. The two went connected at the hip to me. What's more, when I quickly tumbled off track with meal arranging, meal prep went directly alongside it. Actually, however, while the two can live respectively, they don't need to. You can meal prep without making a meal arrangement. (What's more, the other way around!)

Nowadays, in any event, when I don't make a full meal plan, I generally prep a lot of adaptable fixings that can without much of a stretch be transformed into a lot of different meals consistently.

CPSIA information can be obtained
at www.ICGtesting.com
Printed in the USA
BVHW042007250621
610384BV00010B/358